Diabetic*Clarity*

INFORM, PREVENT, AND MAINTAIN

BECOMING MORE INFORMED SO YOU WILL HAVE MORE
CLARITY TO PREVENT AND MAINTAIN DIABETES

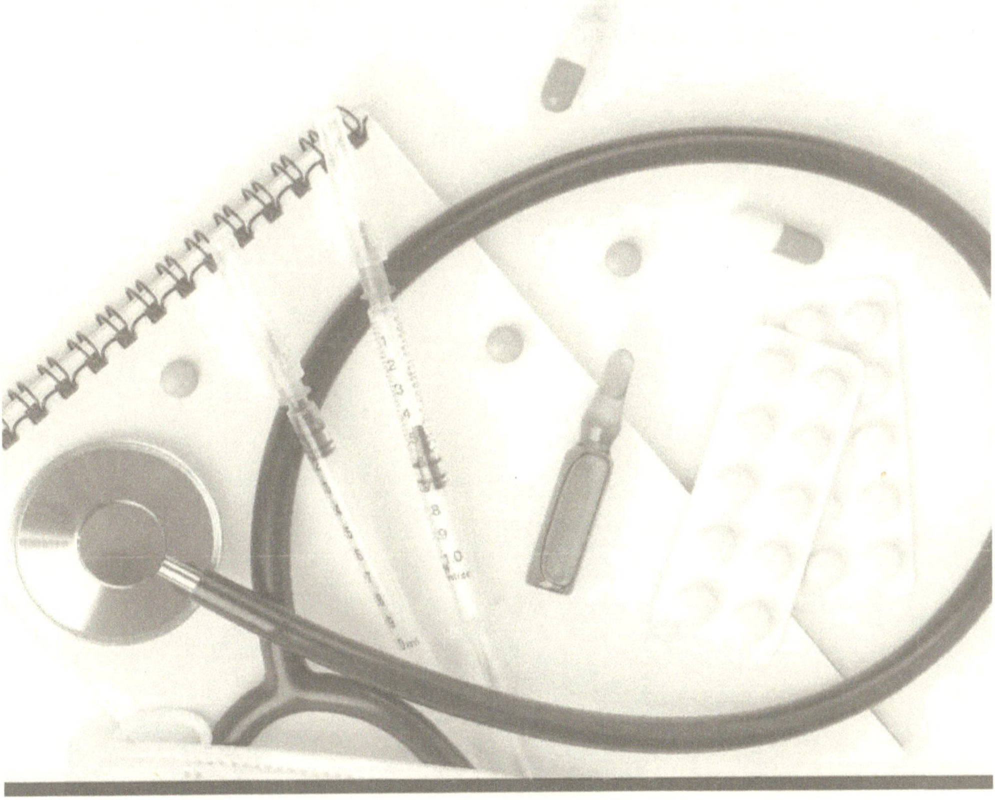

Disclaimer

This e-book has been written for information purposes only. Every effort has been made to make this e-book as complete and accurate as possible.

However, there may be mistakes in typography or content. Also, this e-book provides information only up to the publishing date. Therefore, this e-book should be used as a guide - not as the ultimate source. The purpose of this e-book is to educate. The author and the publisher does not warrant that the information contained in this e-book is fully complete and shall not be responsible for any errors or omissions.

The author and publisher shall have neither liability nor responsibility to any person or entity with respect to any loss or damage caused or alleged to be caused directly or indirectly by this e-book.

DiabeticClarity

INFORM, PREVENT, AND MAINTAIN

Table of Contents

Introduction **7**

    A Look At Type I Diabetes 8

    A Look At Type II Diabetes 8

    A Look At Gestational Diabetes 9

    A Look At Bronze Diabetes 9

    A Look At Diabetes Insipidus 9

Chapter 1: Understanding The Basics Of Diabetes **11**

How Does Diabetes Come About In The First Place? **12**

Chapter 2: Diabetes Symptoms: What Should You Look Out For
.... **14**

The Connection Between Diabetes and Exercise: Why It's So Important?
.... **15**

Chapter 3: How Can Doctors Diagnose and Treat Type 1 and
Type 2 Diabetes **17**

How Do Doctors Diagnose Diabetes? 18

How To Treat Diabetes **19**

How can you effectively manage your blood glucose levels? 19

What Are The Key Points Of Monitoring Your Blood Glucose Levels? 19

Create A Sensible Meal Plan 19

Stay Active With Physical Exercise 20

Taking Medication (Insulin and Diabetes Pills) 21

Why You Need To Self-Monitor Your Blood Sugar Level **21**

What Are The ABCs of Monitoring Your Diabetes? **22**

Chapter 4: What Are The Serious Complications of Out-Of-
Control Diabetes **24**

Diabetic Complications: What Are They and Are They Are Certainty?
.... 25

Poor Oral Health 25

Diabetes Risk Factors 26

What Must Diabetics Understand About Their Condition? **27**

Can You Completely Prevent Diabetes 27

Non-Diabetics 27

Pre-Diabetics 28

Diabetics 28

**Chapter 5: Who Is At Risk For Developing and Living With
Diabetes ....** **29**

What Did The Study Reveal? 30

Yes, Diabetics Can Live A Longer Life 30

Diabetes On Race and Gender **31**

**Chapter 6: The Problems That Affect The Elderly Diabetics and
Their Treatment ....** **33**

Cognitive Dysfunction 34

Functional Impairment 35

Unique Nutritional Needs 35

Why Are Diabetes Symptoms Overlooked In Older Adults? **35**

What Are The Guidelines For Treating Elderly Diabetics? 36

**Chapter 7: How To Come Up With A Workable Diabetic Nutrition
Plan ....** **37**

What Does A Diabetic Nutrition Meal Plan Consists Of? **39**

A Look At The Food Pyramid For Diabetics 39

A Look At Fats and Diabetes **40**

Fiber Can Reduce Your Blood Sugar Level 40

Have Pre-Diabetes? How To Stop It From Worsening **41**

What Is Pre-Diabetes?..41

How Does The Digestive System Work To Break Down Foods and
Drinks?...42

**Chapter 8: What You Can Do To Reverse Your Diabetes
Naturally**...**44**

**10 Ways To Naturally Treat Diabetes (Preventing and Reversing It In
Some Cases)**..**45**

Take Preventive Measures 45

Healthy Diet..45

Add Fiber...46

Add Cinnamon...47

Exercise and Workout Routines 47

Avoid Saturated Fats or Trans Fat Foods..47

Get Control Over Stress 48

Use Nutritional Supplements 48

Eat Smaller Meals...48

Change Your Mindset 48

Conclusion **50**

What's Diabetes Once More? 51

Diabetes' Genetic Factor...52

You Have The Power To Control Your Diabetes..52

Introduction

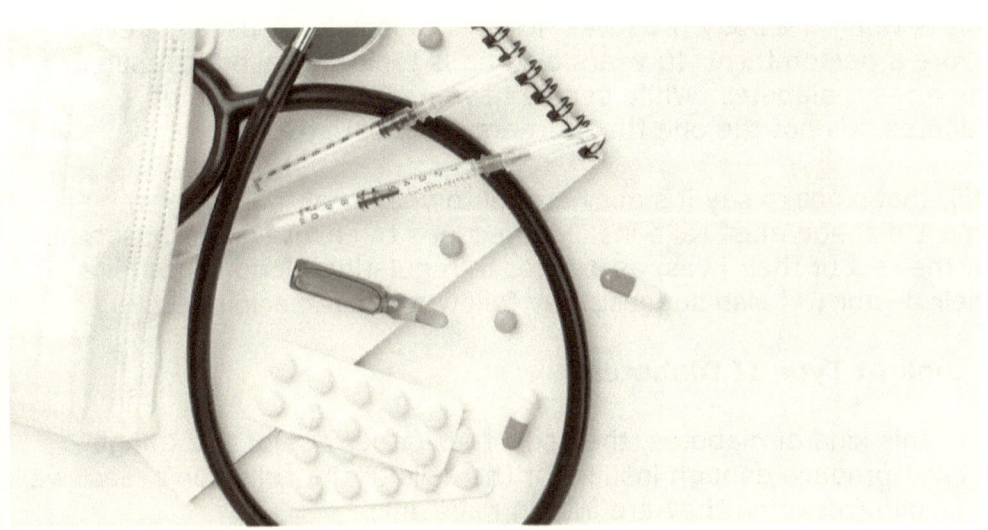

Diabetes Mellitus is the scientific name for the common disease Diabetes.

It's a medical condition where the body's cells cannot take in and use sugar or where there is not enough insulin being secreted into the body. When this happens, the blood sugar level becomes high and stays that way.

The first tale-tell signs of diabetes are the constant need to urinate (or polyuria), constant thirst (or polydipsia) and constant hunger (or polyphagia).

There are five kinds of diabetes, but three common types. They are:

- Type I Diabetes
- Type II Diabetes
- Gestational Diabetes

The rarer types of diabetes are:

- *Bronze Diabetes*

- *Diabetes Insipidus*

A Look At Type I Diabetes

This is when the body produces no level of insulin. It usually develops before a person turns 40 years old and is typically called juvenile or early-onset diabetes. While people have heard of this type of diabetes, it's not the one that garners the most attention.

Still, that's not to say it's not harmful to your health. People who are type 1 diabetic must take insulin injections to ensure sugar absorption for the rest of their lives, as it helps in regulating blood sugar levels. Their doctor will also suggest they follow a strict special diet.

A Look At Type II Diabetes

With this kind of diabetes, the body does either one of two things – doesn't produce enough insulin for the cells or the cells don't react well to insulin (meaning they are insulin resistant).

This is the most common kind of diabetes in the population with nine in every 10 people being type II diabetes.

In order to control this kind of diabetes, you must keep an eye on your blood sugar level, start a weight loss program, make changes to your diet and get lots of exercise.

 These measures, however, will control it – not cure it. When the cells start to weaken and grow, and the immune system doesn't work as good as it used to, your diabetes condition will worsen.

Over time, the patient will need to take start taking insulin in tablet form.

The more you weigh, the higher the chance of developing type II diabetes. Why? Obesity causes the body to secrete chemicals that will weaken the body's cardiovascular and metabolic systems.

However, it's important you understand that obesity isn't the only factor in the development of type II diabetes. If you don't get any kind of exercise and live a sedentary lifestyle, you increase your chances of developing type II diabetes. The wrong foods can also have a negative impact on your lifestyle. Therefore, you need to watch the foods you consume.

A Look At Gestational Diabetes

This diabetes type is seen only in pregnant women. It occurs when a woman has an excessive amount of blood glucose and the body cannot generate enough insulin to use all the sugar. When gestational diabetes isn't controlled, it can result in childbirth complications.

The baby may be bigger than they should be, which means the woman may need a C-section. Once gestational diabetes is diagnosed, the woman must start using blood-sugar controlling medications.

According to various research, consuming a significant amount of cholesterol and animal fat increases a woman's chance of developing gestational diabetes. If you plan on becoming pregnant, you must control how much animal fat and cholesterol you consume.

A Look At Bronze Diabetes

Bronze diabetes – also called hemochromatosis – is diagnosed when doctors note the body is absorbing a significant amount of iron from the food you consume. The name comes from what it does to the body – darkens the skin and hyperglycemia.

This type of diabetes is the result of a faulty gene and will eventually lead to potential damage in other bodily organs. Due to the fact that bronze diabetes can cause damage to organs, a liver biopsy must be done to see if damage has taken place.

Bronze diabetes symptoms tend to become noticeable at age 40. Doctors will diagnose people with this condition by doing a serum ferritin and transferrin saturation blood test. It may also be necessary to do a DNA blood test to see if it's genetic.

A Look At Diabetes Insipidus

This is a rare diabetes type, which results in the imbalance of bodily fluids. Due to the imbalance, you may still be thirsty even if you just drank something. Due to the excess amount of water or beverage you drink, you're liable to urinate more often.

Diabetes Insipidus, like type 1 diabetes, has no cure, but there are treatments doctors can recommend that alleviate your constant need to drink and reduce how many times you run to the bathroom.

This condition occurs when the body cannot balance its fluid level, but the health problems you can have from it depend on the kind of diabetes insipidus you have:

- Central diabetes insipidus
- Nephrogenic diabetes insipidus
- Gestational diabetes insidious
- Primary polydipsia

A doctor will often diagnose a person with this condition by the symptoms of constant urination and the excessive need to drink.

While gestational diabetes, bronze diabetes and diabetes insipidus are important, they are not as common as types 1 and 2.

For the purpose of this e-book, you will learn more about type 1 and type 2 diabetes – how they develop, how you can control them, what their symptoms are, how to live healthy with the conditions and how to naturally reverse type 2 diabetes.

Chapter 1: Understanding The Basics Of Diabetes

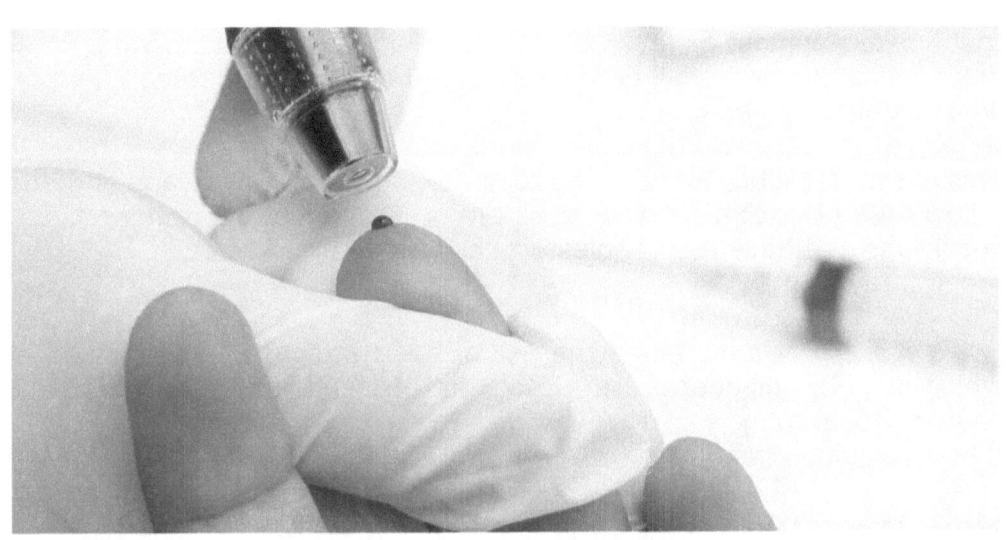

You've heard of the term "diabetes" and have a general understanding of what the disease is.

It's a disease in which the blood glucose levels are higher than they should be. Special Note: Glucose also means sugar. The condition develops because the sugar cannot get into the cells, which means they starve for sugar.

Think of it as a person being around all the good food, but the mouth is sewn shut and they are unable to eat – pretty much the same thing.

There are an estimated 17 million Americans who have diabetes with one-third who don't even realize they have the disease. That's a real problem!

After all, diabetes can lead to an array of health problems, including but not limited to:

- Blindness

- Heart disease
- Kidney failure
- Amputations in the lower extremities (think toes, feet and legs)

In just the U.S., diabetes is the sixth leading cause of death, and that's because most have developed heart disease. A person with diabetes as the same risk of having a heart attack as a person who has already had one.

This is why diabetics are advised to speak with their physicians and follow their physician's advice at all times. They must get regular check-ups and have their cholesterol and blood pressured monitored often.

Using tobacco also increases the risk of heart attacks in diabetics, which is why diabetics are urged to quit smoking or doing chewing tobacco.

How Does Diabetes Come About In The First Place?

Understand, there are five kinds of diabetes, but the basic premise of the disease is the same. Whatever type of diabetes a person has, the key reason for the development is that the body cannot produce or use glucose effectively.

When this happens, it causes the body's blood sugar levels to rise and stay above the normal range.

There are three things you should understand:

- The body's cells, which uses the glucose, need to absorb the sugar in the blood so it can be turned into fuel.

- The insulin, produced by the ever-important pancreas organ, will let the sugar get into the cells.

- The glucose that's broken down from food, liver or muscles, is known as glycogen.

Consider diabetes as being your car's locking gas cap. If you understand the way this cap works, you have a good idea of how diabetes works. The cells have this locking gas cap, and the insulin is what happens the locking gas cap, and the glucose is the gas for the car.

In other types of diabetes, the body produces the insulin but not enough for the body. A minute number of the cells will allow the glucose to come through. Another problem is that some cells won't work as they should and don't allow the glucose to come in.

Every one of these is a recipe for a copious amount of glucose in the bloodstream.

Chapter 2: Diabetes Symptoms: What Should You Look Out For

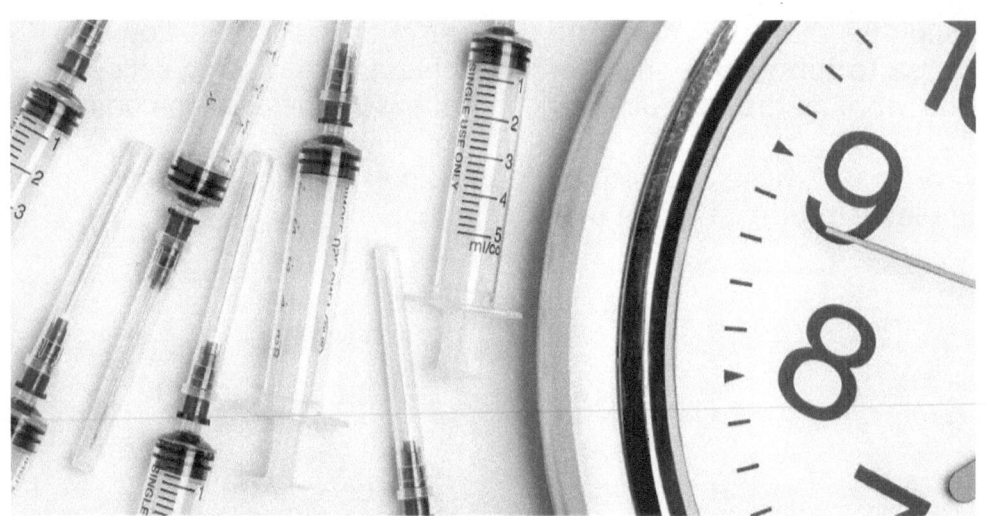

People who believe they have diabetics must visit their doctor to get an official diagnosis.

If you have any of the following symptoms, it's imperative you see your doctor right away: extreme thirst, constant urination, excessive hunger, numbness or tingling in the extremities, excessive tiredness, slow healing sores, dry skin, reoccurring infections, unexplained weight loss, vomiting, stomach pains and nausea.

Most people are under the mistaken impression that since glucose is sugar all they need to do is stop eating sweets. Wrong!

The reality is that the majority of foods and the carbohydrates eaten break down into a simple structure called glucose. When the food hits the stomach, the stomach immediately begins breaking down the food.

The stomach breaks the carbohydrates down for the glucose while the proteins are broken down for the amino acids. Once the food is broken down, the body uses it for other things. The blood will pick it up, so the cells can use it for energy.

For healthy people, the blood picks the glucose that's been absorbed in the GI tract up and lets the pancreas know that it needs to produce and release insulin. In type II diabetes, the body doesn't produce enough of the insulin or the cells are unable to take in the insulin.

For both cases, the cells don't receive the glucose needed for energy, which leaves the glucose to float throughout the bloodstream. When there is a build-up of glucose in the body, it leads to blood vessel and organ damage, increasing your chances of heart disease.

It's vitally important for you to maintain normal-to-close-to normal glucose levels. When there is a high level of glucose, it starts to spill over into the urine.

The Connection Between Diabetes and Exercise: Why It's So Important?

There are 21 million people in the U.S. who have diabetes with another 6.2 million oblivious to the fact that they have the disease.

Based on information from the American Diabetes Association, people who have diabetes pay 2.3 times more in medical expenses than people without diabetes. The Population Health Management believes diabetes costs the healthcare industry $218 billion.

However, the majority of diabetes cases can be prevented through a healthy lifestyle – exercise and diet.

Of course, you have to take that in for a minute – 6.2 million people don't know they have diabetes and 57 million people with pre-diabetes. If the pre-diabetics knew how to take care of their health, then they may never develop type 2 diabetes.

A person who is pre-diabetic can stop themselves from getting full-blown type II diabetes. By losing weight and increasing exercise, you can reverse the damage and bring the glucose back to normal.

This is what most people don't understand – a proper diet and exercise can stop a person from developing diabetes.

What are the signs of diabetes? You may see signs of diabetes in your family and friends without even realizing it. It's possible that people you know are diabetic and don't even know it.

The Center for Disease Control and Prevention believes one in three Americans will get diabetes at some point in their life – staggering numbers if you really think about it.

What about those Type 2 diabetics that are diagnosed with their condition? Would they change their ways if they knew diet and exercise could reverse the disease?

Of course, to have all this, it means dismissing the myths and beliefs that impede their chances. The drug companies don't want diabetics to know that diet and exercise plays a huge role in reversing Type II diabetes.

The healthcare system is in real trouble – the nation is in trouble. This is why it's important for people to start to take personal responsibility for their health.

Many people who understand what diabetes still have questions about their health such as:

- Should they be reducing their sugar intake?
- Is the weight increasing their risk?
- If they are skinny, does this lower their risk?
- Are diet and exercise so important?
- How can blood sugar levels be controlled?

Bear in mind that are some issues that people have no idea what to ask? For example,

- A person who has diabetes for over five years has increased their chances of developing cardiovascular disease.
- Getting regular exercise can increase insulin sensitivity, which allows you to alleviate your medication dosages.

Chapter 3: How Can Doctors Diagnose and Treat Type 1 and Type 2 Diabetes

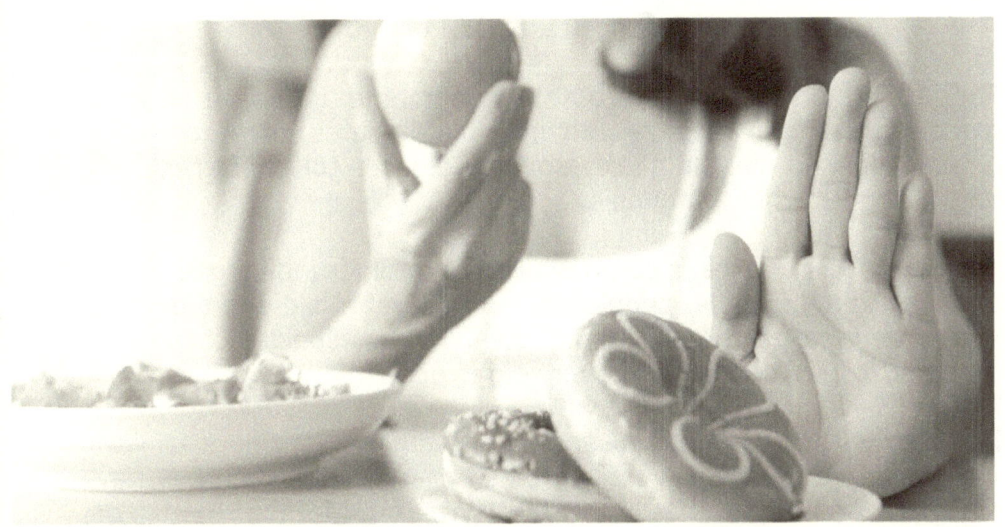

Diabetes is considered to be the "silent" disease because most people show little to no symptoms or signs of having it.

These symptoms include:

- Constant urination
- Excessive hunger
- Excessive thirst
- Unexplained weight loss
- Slow healing sores
- Dry, itchy skin
- Tingling feet
- Blurry sight

Unfortunately, there are too many people who have diabetes and never show any signs.

Type II diabetes symptoms gradually appear while type 1 diabetes quickly develop.

How Do Doctors Diagnose Diabetes?

Doctors will use all kinds of tests to diagnose diabetes, including:

- Fasting plasma glucose (FPG) test
- Oral glucose tolerance test (OGTT)

The random plasma glucose test lets doctors learn if their patients has diabetes. If any test reveals possible diabetes, the doctor will do a repeat fasting plasma glucose or oral glucose tolerance test another day to confirm their diagnosis.

Since type II diabetes is commonly seen in older individuals and overweight individuals, people who are 45 years old and older should be tested annually for diabetes. This is especially true if a person is older than 45 and overweight/obese.

Diabetes is a very serious disease that leads to disability, pain and death – some people have symptoms but never suspect they have diabetes. And, since they don't feel symptomatic, they never get a check-up.

Although there is a risk for diabetes due to weight and age, people never get tested. And, undiagnosed diabetes can lead to serious health complications such as death.

Most times, people don't get diagnosed until they suffer from the other serious health problems such as difficulty seeing, blurriness and heart problems.

However, with regular check-ups and early detection, you can stop the complications before they occur.

How To Treat Diabetes

Diabetes has no known cure, but by carefully monitoring blood glucose, blood pressure and cholesterol levels, the disease can be well-managed.

Type I diabetics must take insulin injections – through an insulin pump or shots – to keep control over the blood glucose levels. Type II diabetics will need to use insulin, oral medications or a combination of both to control their glucose levels.

However, type II diabetics can reverse their condition by following a healthy diet and exercise routine.

How can you effectively manage your blood glucose levels?

- Create and follow a meal plan that is sensible for you, listening to how your body responds to the foods you consume.
- Add more physical activity to your everyday life
- Use your doctor-prescribed medication and continually check your blood glucose levels based on the doctor's recommendations.

What Are The Key Points Of Monitoring Your Blood Glucose Levels?

Create A Sensible Meal Plan

To ensure your blood glucose levels stay within the normal range, you must make good healthy food choices. Diabetics must have a well-thought-out meal plan that is based on how their body responds to the foods consumed.

This can be achieved by seeking out the assistance of a diabetes teacher, dietician or nutritionist.

When you're creating your meal plan, you need to remember a few factors:

- Weight

- Blood glucose levels
- Medications
- Physical activity

With the meal plan, you can attain a healthy weight, which will help you to gain control over your blood glucose levels. With the assistance of a dietician, you'll learn about the myths of healthy eating and ensure that you and your family can follow a plan that meets your lifestyle.

Diabetics can eat food that is good for anyone to eat – foods that are low in salt, sugar and fat and high in fiber like beans, fruits, vegetables and whole grains.

With healthy choices, you can maintain a healthy weight that controls the blood glucose levels and decreases the chance for heart disease.

Stay Active With Physical Exercise

It is imperative that diabetics lead a physically active lifestyle. According to research, older adults who regularly exercise tend to have better glucose levels. And, there is a reason for that.

Exercise provides an array of health benefits that people with diabetes need to focus on getting. You can attain a healthy weight, improve insulin function to reduce their blood glucose level, improve their heart and lungs and boost their energy levels.

Of course, before you can start an exercise regime, you should speak with your doctor. Some exercises may not be safe. For example, it's not advised for people who have high blood pressure or eye problems to lift weights.

Let your doctor give you a physical check-up and let you know what physical activity is best for you. Your doctor can recommend exercises that can help reduce the weight and keep your blood sugar levels under control.

It's important to take part in physical activity every day. Go walking or biking. You can also do some gardening. You can partake in swimming and dancing or just stay active around the house doing chores such as cleaning the bathroom or kitchen.

There are all kinds of activities that you can do every day to increase your physical prowess. The key is to get 30 minutes of exercise each day. Again, if you've not exercised in some time (or ever), be sure to slowly increase how often you exercise as well as its intensity.

Taking Medication (Insulin and Diabetes Pills)

Type 1 diabetics and some type II diabetics will need to use insulin to reduce their blood sugar levels. People using insulin, which is a liquid hormone, are doing so because the body doesn't generate enough of it. It's usually given by insulin pump or shot.

Most type II diabetics can take diabetes pills because the body generates the insulin but is unable to use it properly.

The doctor will determine how the medication is taken, but make sure that any side affects you notice are reported to your doctor. The diabetes pill is not a substitute for a healthy lifestyle but in addition to your healthy regime.

There are cases where some type II diabetics never need either one but follow a healthy diet and get regular amounts of exercise to treat the condition.

Why You Need To Self-Monitor Your Blood Sugar Level

A blood glucose monitor can help you to monitor your blood glucose levels.

Be sure to log these readings in a diary to get a good idea of how the treatment is going. You can do this multiple time a day or once a day – the choice is really up to you and your doctor.

With constant monitoring, you can identify the highs and lows of your blood sugar levels. Hypoglycemia is when the blood glucose level is too low.

A hypoglycemic person may come across as altered and shaky. A decreased level of blood glucose may lead to fainting. However, following the doctor-prescribed treatment plan and constant monitoring of your blood sugar levels will help you to avoid these lows.

Be sure to check the level. If you find it's too low, you can increase it by eating or drinking something sugary such as fruit juice or peanut butter.

Hyperglycemia is when the glucose levels are too high. If the blood glucose is higher than normal, a person could go into a diabetic coma. Continually experiencing highs means an adjustment must be made to the plan previously laid out.

What Are The ABCs of Monitoring Your Diabetes?

Diabetics are at significant risk of suffering from strokes or having heart disease.

That's why you need to remember the ABC of blood glucose monitoring. They are:

- AIC (average blood glucose)
- Blood pressure
- Cholesterol

The AIC test gives you a good idea of what the blood glucose level is the majority of the time. A test result of less than seven is a good sign that you have your diabetes under control.

Anything more than that means your levels are too high. If they're too high, you must speak with your doctor about a new treatment plan and lifestyle that will help you get control over your diabetes.

By lowering your AIC levels to a good level, you can lower your chances of complications tied to diabetes (kidney damage or heart disease).

High blood pressure leads to an array of complications such as kidney disease, stroke and other health problems. Diabetics should keep their blood pressure within the 130/80 or lower range.

Be sure your doctor checks your blood pressure every time you visit. If the reading is too high, the doctor may suggest ways to reduce it.

Cholesterol, such as LDL cholesterol, is a fat-like substance that accumulates in the arteries. If your doctor notices the cholesterol levels are excessively high, it means the arteries are narrowed.

This can cause a person to suffer from heart disease or have a heart attack. Diabetics need to have a cholesterol level of 100 or less. Any time your cholesterol level is higher than this, it's important to redefine the treatment plan that will lower it.

Chapter 4: What Are The Serious Complications of Out-Of-Control Diabetes

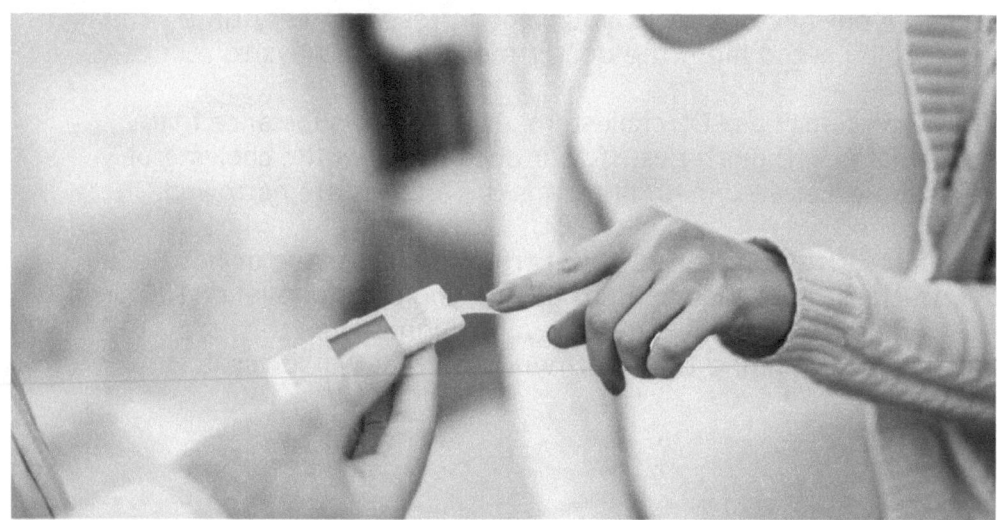

There are so many hidden dangers associated with diabetes – before the diagnosis and afterward if the condition is left untreated.

Its why diabetes has become known as the silent killer. According to various statistics, there are about 18 million type 1 and type 2 diabetics living in the U.S. – that's not including pregnant women with gestational diabetes or the other kinds of diabetes people can suffer from.

Most people, diabetics too, have no inkling of how dangerous their disease can be. Would it surprise you to know that diabetics will die – on average – 10 years earlier than people without diabetes?

Why the shorter lifespans though – even if they are taking good care of themselves? This is a not-so-easy answer, but it all boils down to the complications diabetes patients tend to have.

Diabetic Complications: What Are They and Are They Are Certainty?

In short, these are chronic health conditions that affect a diabetic's body. These conditions are the result of a condition doctors have dubbed "Advanced Glycation End products" where an excessive amount of sugar gets into the cells.

AGE can cause problems such as:

- Vascular disease
- Coronary artery disease
- Kidney disease
- Blindness
- Peripheral neuropathy (loss of feeling in extremities)
- Retinopathy (blindness)

Poor Oral Health

Another, not-so-widely known complication of diabetes is poor oral health. When you have diabetes, you are more susceptible to mouth problems such as cavities and dry mouth. This can cause ulcers to develop too.

Gingivitis is another oral health issue, which can be identified by red, swollen and bleeding gums. It develops because the mouth is unable to get rid of the foods and bacteria (dry mouth).

Diabetes can also cause mouth infections. While most people view infections as being bacterial, they can also be fungal such as thrush or a yeast infection. Sugar thrives on people who have uncontrolled or undiagnosed diabetes.

Another serious oral health problem diabetics have is periodontitis, which an infection that affects the mouth's supporting structures like bone ligaments. With this gum infection, you could lose your teeth early in life or suffer from gum abscess due to the lack of collagen in the mouth.

The real problem about diabetes is that, in most cases, it's not diagnosed until it's too late. That's because there are no noticeable symptoms in the disease's early stages. With untreated (undiagnosed) diabetes, these complications can get some traction because of AGE. And, statistics demonstrate that more than five million people have diabetes but do not even know it.

The general consensus about diabetic complications is given time, and uncontrolled diabetes will lead to complications. The longer the diabetic does not know or take care of themselves, the higher the chances for complications to ensue. How well a person controls their sugar level will dictate their complication risk.

When the body is constantly hit by highs and lows of sugar, it puts pressure on the cells, nerves, veins, arteries and capillaries. This will lead to complications.

However, by maintaining constant control over blood sugar levels and staying active physically, you lower the chance of diabetes-related complications.

Diabetes Risk Factors

A person considered to be pre-diabetic can go into full-blown diabetes if they have any of the following factors:

- Overweight/obese
- Family history of diabetes
- Lack of exercise
- History of gestational diabetes
- Ethnicity

People 45 and older with any of the above risk factors need to be screened annually – your yearly medical exam. According to statistics, these individuals make up most of the diabetes diagnosed cases every year.

Doctors will use two tests to diagnose a person with diabetes:

- Fasting plasma glucose test
- Oral glucose tolerance test

Both tests will demonstrate the body's glucose intolerance – where the blood sugar is considered higher than what is deemed normal. Of course, this is no real indication of actual diabetes.

What Must Diabetics Understand About Their Condition?

Diabetics must always be mindful of their lifestyle – how active they are and what foods they eat. By doing this, they can reduce their chances of suffering from diabetes-related complications for quite some time.

A person who eats a proper diet, exercises regularly, gets the right amount of sleep and maintains control over their blood sugar levels can improve their quality of life significantly.

They will also live a much longer and healthier life than a person with diabetes who is not taking proper care of themselves and their diet.

A diabetic will develop complications if they allow their diabetes to stay high over a period of weeks. They could become blind, suffer from an amputation, be unable to move and care for themselves or even die due to a heart attack.

While this seems like a grim outcome for diabetics, the reality is that changes your lifestyle and diet can prevent them.

According to research, diabetics who maintain controlled sugar levels and follow a good, healthy diet are able to stave off diabetes-related complications and develop fewer, if any, of the complications than people who refuse to make the necessary changes in their life.

Can You Completely Prevent

Diabetes Non-Diabetics

If you're not yet diagnosed with diabetes (have sugar levels within the normal range), taking good care of yourself by eating healthy and getting exercise are the primary ways in which never to develop diabetes. If you are at risk for developing the disease, you need to make necessary lifestyle changes:

- Avoid eating refined carbs and sugars
- Limit your sugar consumption (no sodas, cakes and candy every day)
- Increase your activity level (join a gym, walk the mall or neighborhood, etc.)
- Lose weight if overweight or obese (According to research, a minute amount of weight loss can do the body a world of good in terms of good health.)

Pre-Diabetics

A person who is classified as pre-diabetic needs to really watch their diet more carefully. For this reason, they need to seek the advice of a healthcare professional and/or dietician to learn what foods they need to avoid and limit their consumption of cookies, cakes and other sugar-laden foods.

Pre-diabetics are advised to eat smaller, more nutritious meals (five small meals rather than three big ones).

Diabetics

People who have diabetes – full-blown diabetes – must take great care of their health and follow their doctor's advice.

They need to see a doctor regularly to have their eyes, blood pressure, blood sugar and cholesterol checked. Uncontrolled diabetes is responsible for tens of thousands of deaths every year.

It's up to diabetics to not become a part of that statistic.

Chapter 5: Who Is At Risk For Developing and Living With Diabetes

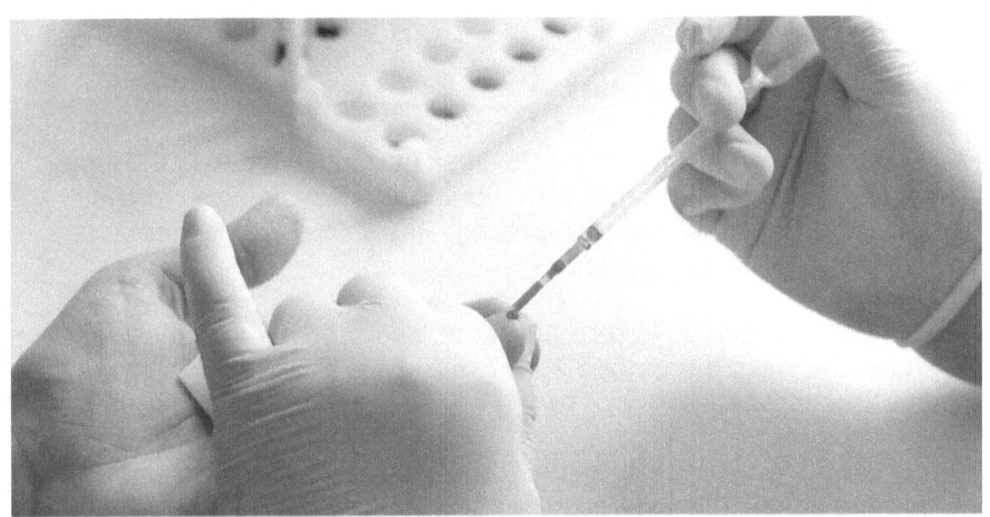

According to the well-known international medical journal, Lancet, the number of Americans at risk for developing diabetes is rapidly rising.

However, the journal's study also revealed the risks of developing diabetes was dependent on three things:

- Race
- Education
- Geographical location

This is the first stay in over 10 years about the risks people in the U.S. face in developing diabetes. The U.S. Center for Disease Control and Prevention epidemiologists have been keeping track and reviewing how prevalent diabetes is and how many new cases are being reported every year.

The researchers looked at the mortality data of 600,000 people from 1985 to 2011 to look at the risks of the common kinds of diabetes – type 1 and 2 – and excluded the others – gestational diabetes, bronze diabetes and diabetes insipidus.

While the study looked at the disease in American people, it's liable the results would have been similar for other parts of the world if European data has been used where a Western diet and lifestyle is normal.

What Did The Study Reveal?

Based on the information for the 25-year period, there was a huge spike in the number of people who would develop diabetes in their lifetime. In 1985, girls were 27 percent likely to develop diabetes whereas boys had a 21 percent.

In 2011, this number spiked to 40 percent for both genders. Therefore, the risks have doubled for the boys, and the girls saw a 50 percent increase.

There was no look into why this study revealed such a dramatic increase. However, it's believed that people who have diabetes have longer lifespans, which increases the chances of developing diabetes in their lifetime.

Yes, Diabetics Can Live A Longer Life

Even if you're diagnosed with diabetes, your lifespan isn't dramatically shortened if you take good care of yourself. U.S. children with diabetes can live another good 70 years with their disease with a good sensible diet and exercise routine.

For the 25-year period (1985 to 2011), the years, men who were diagnosed with diabetes were expected to survive with an increase of 156 percent. Women only had a 70 percent increase.

No answers as to why the difference, but it's thought that medical advancements such as knowledge and treatments are the reason.

However, having diabetes does shorten one's lifespan. During this period, researchers noted there was 46 percent of men, and 44 percent of women died from diabetic complication.

This is mainly because of the rise of diabetes itself and fewer cases of diabetes being diagnosed and untreated.

Despite the whole diabetes picture looking grim, the truth is that the individual diabetic is actually seeing improvements.

Both men and women who are diabetic are likely to live two years more than in times' past – perhaps the result is from better treatment options and plans.

Diabetes On Race and Gender

Overall, Americans have a grim 40 percent of being diagnosed with diabetes, but for Hispanics and blacks, the percentages are even worse.

- For whites – 37 percent of white boys and 34 percent of white girls will develop diabetes.
- For blacks – 44.7 percent of black men and 55.3 percent of black women will develop the disease.
- For Hispanics – 51.8 percent of Hispanic males and 51.5 percent of Hispanic women will develop diabetes.

If anything, this strengthens the argument that diabetes has a genetic role in who does and does not develop the disease. This means your genes can predispose you to the disease.

Still, the majority of medical researchers agree that lifestyle plays a huge role in its development.

Researchers looked at race because they had the information available, but they agree that socio-economic status is just as important as race – maybe even more so.

Whatever the reason, white people are far less likely to be diagnosed as diabetic then blacks and Hispanics. Both races are 50 percent more likely than whites to be diagnosed with diabetes.

However, researchers are still trying to determine why black men are 10 percent less likely to develop the disease than black women. Genetic differences cannot be explained, and the jury is still out on why this happens.

Chapter 6: The Problems That Affect The Elderly Diabetics and Their Treatment

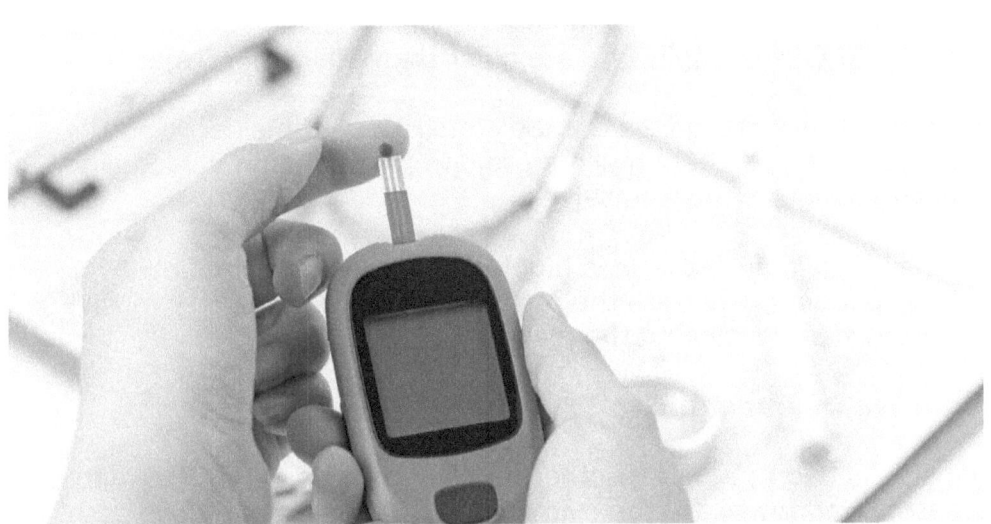

A person who has been diagnosed with diabetes needs to take very good care of themselves, but this can be much harder for an elderly patient to do for various other reasons including but not limited to:

- Home situation
- Cognitive abilities
- Comorbidities
- Other medications

Of course, as older adults with diabetes, the importance of their health needs to focus on nutrition and avoid becoming hypoglycemic. After all, as people age, they don't eat near as often, putting them at risk for malnutrition and hypoglycemia.

Now, most diabetes-treatment guidelines are geared toward people in their middle ages with the same recommendations for everybody –

young and old. However, it's important that elderly diabetics get an individualized plan that's tailored to their particular situation.

The life expectancy for a man in the U.S. is 88 years old while the life expectancy for a U.S. female is 90 years old.

People classify the elderly into two categories:

- Young-Old – Those who are between 65 and 80 years of age.
- Old-Old – People who are older than 80 years of age.

Of course, these categories are too simplistic to the elderly, and diabetes can affect them much more differently than a person who is much younger than themselves.

Since an individualized plan is highly recommended for older diabetic patients, what are the primary issues that a doctor must consider when developing the plan?

Cognitive Dysfunction

Diabetes is tied to a host of other medical conditions for older adults. Geriatric syndromes are the culmination of various conditions such as cognitive dysfunction, functional impairment and others. These conditions can affect how well a person with diabetes can care for themselves.

Cognitive dysfunction such as Alzheimer's disease, dementia and others are two times more likely to affect a person with diabetes. These conditions can range from subtleness to complete memory loss.

This means a person who has diabetes and a decline in their cognitive abilities will be unable to properly care for themselves such as testing, changing doses of insulin and taking care of their diet.

For that reason, older diabetic patient caregivers are advised to keep constant track of the diabetes patient and monitor their blood sugar levels to reduce the chance for hypoglycemia.

Functional Impairment

Another problem is their functional impairment. Older diabetics tend to be less active and suffer from more functional impairment. They may have difficulty with hearing and seeing, may have balance issues, suffer from peripheral neuropathy (loss of feeling in their extremities) and so much more.

These problems can limit a diabetic from getting the physical activity they need to stay healthy and keep their blood sugar down.

Unique Nutritional Needs

The nutritional needs of older diabetic patients are especially important (though it's important for any diabetes patient regardless of their age). As a person ages, their energy needs begin to drop, but the macronutrient needs stay the same.

It can be very difficult to meet these micronutrient needs if a person isn't consuming enough calories. It's not uncommon for older adults to suffer from swallowing difficulties, anorexia, altered tastes and others.

This is why doctors are advised to create a Mini-Nutritional Assessment for older adults with diabetes either with the patient or with their caregiver and a nutritionist.

The plan needs to take into consideration goals, preferences, their culture and abilities.

These are just three of the many things doctors with older diabetic patients need to consider when treating their patients.

Why Are Diabetes Symptoms Overlooked In Older Adults?

Many of the classic symptoms of diabetes such as tingling hands or fingers, blurry vision, weight loss, slow healing wounds, etc. are overlooked in the elderly as just a sign of getting older.

Too many doctors are all too dismissive of these and other symptoms and don't test their elderly patients for diabetes. It's not until it's almost too late that doctors notice something is amiss and step in to control the problem.

What Are The Guidelines For Treating Elderly Diabetics?

There have been a few organizations that have developed elderly diabetic guidelines. In the yearly Standards of Medical Care in Diabetes, there is a section targeted for older adults, with recommendations as follows:

Older diabetic patients who can still function - cognitively and actively – with a good life expectancy can follow the diabetic care that has been developed for younger adult diabetics.

Older adults who glycemic goals have not been made may need an individualized care plan but making sure that no hyperglycemia symptoms complications can develop.

The treatment of older diabetic adults with cardiovascular risk factors should be based on how long the benefit would be and the patient themselves.

The majority of older adults have hypertension (high blood pressure) and can use an aspirin or lipid therapy to boost their life expectancy so long as it equals the primary or secondary prevention therapy's timeframe.

Older diabetic adults need to be screened regularly for diabetes complications, paying special mind to the complications that could affect them functionally and cognitively.

Chapter 7: How To Come Up With A Workable Diabetic Nutrition Plan

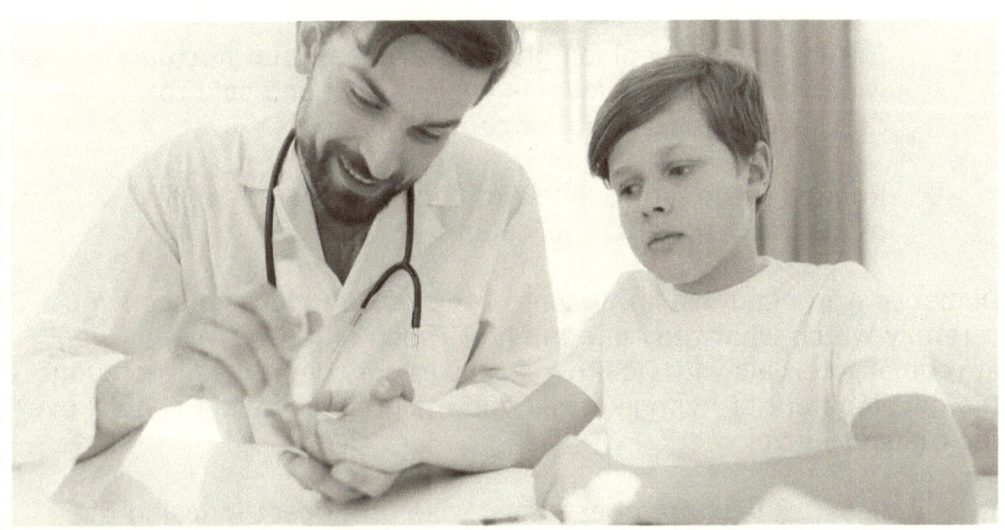

The groundwork of any diabetes management plan is to focus on weight control, diet and good nutrition.

Of all plans created, controlling diabetes means controlling how much food you consume, so you maintain a good weight and keep your blood sugar level stable. It's not easy to get control over your bad habits, but it's a way to reverse type 2 diabetes. Why is it so difficult?

The nutritional aspects of diabetes are complex, which is why you should always consult with a registered nutritionist or dietician to develop a sensible diabetic nutrition plan.

Any plan you develop should be based on goals as laid out by the American Diabetes Association and its Evidence-Based Nutrition Principles and Recommendations for Treatment and Prevention of Diabetes and Related Complications.

What are these goals?

- Ensure that all important food requirements are met such as vitamins and minerals.

- Ensure that all energy needs are met.

- Ensure that a reasonable weight is attained and maintained.

- Ensure that daily blood glucose levels are not fluctuating widely and that the level is near normal and safe to decrease the possibility of complications.

- Reduce serum lipids levels to decrease the possibility of macro-vascular complication.

Diabetics who need insulin to control their blood glucose levels must carefully watch what they eat and how much of it. They need to eat at regular intervals with healthy snacks in between times to prevent the development of hypoglycemia and maintain complete control over their glucose level.

Type 2 diabetics who are obese must take great care in losing the weight. Since obesity can cause insult resistance, people may need oral anti-diabetic agents or insulin to control how much glucose stays in the bloodstream.

By losing weight, they may be able to stop the need for medication. Even a minute weight loss of 10 percent can do wonders for the body and blood sugar levels.

Even if one is not using insulin to control their diabetes, eat regular, but smaller meals and regular intervals can help reduce the weight. Nobody needs to skip a meal, but diabetics most certainly should never skip them. The key is to pace the food out so that the pancreas as more manageable demands put on it.

The biggest challenge of dealing with diabetes is adhering to a long-term diabetes meal plan. Obese diabetics have a little easier time in that all they need to do is moderately restrict their calorie intake.

People who are maintaining their weight may find this a bit trickier. For them, they need to be willing to instill need dietary habits into their lifestyle, educate themselves about food and diabetes, take part in behavioral therapy, join a support group and get constant nutrition counseling.

What Does A Diabetic Nutrition Meal Plan Consists Of?

Every diabetic nutrition meal plan will not be the same, as it's based on five key things:

- Lifestyle
- Food preferences
- Cultural background
- Ethnic background
- Normal eating times

People who are doing insulin therapy have some flexibility in their meals' content and timing, as they can adjust their insulin dosage to correlate with their lifestyle – exercise and diet.

Thanks to the progress in insulin management, it's allowed people to take advantage of the flexible schedule. In the past, people had to adjust their schedule to meet the insulin duration and actions.

To create a workable meal plan, a detailed diet history must be taken. This will help to look at eating habits and lifestyle. An assessment of weight gain, loss or maintenance will also be done. It's not unusual for people with type 2 diabetics to be overweight and need to lose weight.

A Look At The Food Pyramid For Diabetics

Another great way to come up with a meal plan is to review the Diabetic Meal Plan. This is especially helpful for people with type 2 diabetes who have a problem with controlling the number of calories they consume.

There are six food groups on the Diabetic Food Pyramid:

- Grains, breads and starches
- Vegetables (non-starchy vegetables)
- Fruits
- Milk products
- Meat and other proteins
- Fats, sweets and oils

How much should a diabetic consume from each of the food groups? The key is to consume 50 to 60 percent of their calories from the fruits, vegetables and starches. The higher in the pyramid, the less food you should consume from them.

The top of the pyramid – fats, sweets and oils – should be consumed sporadically. By doing so, diabetics can gain control over their blood sugar levels and reach a healthier weight while also reducing their chance of cardiovascular disease.

A Look At Fats and Diabetes

Diabetics are encouraged to reduce how many calories they consume from fat – less than 30 percent is ideal. They also need to reduce saturated fats to 10 percent.

Total dietary cholesterol should be under 30mg per day. By doing this, diabetics decrease numerous risk factors like high serum cholesterol levels that can lead to coronary heart disease – the number one cause of death for diabetics.

Make sure your diabetic meal plan consists of non-animal protein sources (peanut butter, for example). However, if there are any signs of renal disease, diabetics are encouraged to reduce their protein consumption amount.

Fiber Can Reduce Your Blood Sugar Level

Diabetics are encouraged to increase their consumption of fiber, as a high-fiber diet can help in reducing total cholesterol and low-density lipoprotein cholesterol.

It can help with reducing the need for exogenous insulin and better the blood glucose level.
There are two kinds of fiber:

- **Soluble** – These are found in foods such as oat, legumes and some fruit. When combined with water, it creates a gel that causes the stomach's content to leave the digestive tract slowly. It's thought that this fiber can also slow the glucose absorption rate.

- **Insoluble fiber** – These are found in whole grain cereals, breads and certain vegetables, which can increase the amount of stool and stop constipation.

The biggest issue with fiber consumption is that diabetics may need to adjust their insulin dosage to stop hypoglycemia from happening.

Make sure to steadily increase the consumption of fiber to avoid any complications and talk with a dietician.

Have Pre-Diabetes? How To Stop It From Worsening

Millions of people all around the world are suffering from diabetes. Diabetics who fail to control their blood sugar levels can suffer from even more serious medical conditions such as kidney failure, nerve damage, heart disease, etc.

What Is Pre-Diabetes?

This is the condition where the body's blood glucose levels are higher than normal but not so high to be considered a diabetic. According to various research, 70 percent of people who are classified as pre-diabetic become actual diabetics with type II diabetes.

Consider that just for a moment – 70 percent of all people with pre-diabetes become type II diabetics, which means 30 percent of individuals are able to stop the condition from becoming chronic. Pre-diabetes does not mean full-blown diabetes.

While you can't change the past, your age or genes, you can change the way you live – what kinds of foods and drinks you consume.

How Does The Digestive System Work To Break Down Foods and Drinks?

The foods you consume are a combination of fats, carbohydrates and proteins. For example, meat is a mixture of protein and fats, while vegetables and fruits are filled with carbohydrates.

When the body begins to digest the food, it's broken down into three key parts – carbs, fats and proteins. They are then broken down, even more, released into the bloodstream and delivered throughout the body.

The energy your body needs comes from glucose, which is a simple sugar. However, it's the body's main energy source. The majority of glucose is generated from the carb's starch and sugar seen in breads, fruits, grains, pasts, potatoes, rice and more.

The digestive process produces the glucose that then gets absorbed into the bloodstream and is sent to the cells.

Glucose is the cell's fuel, giving your body its movements, its brain the power to think and so much more. The only way the cells can get their power is through insulin's help.

Insulin is a chemical hormone that the pancreas produces. When this happens, the insulin flows through the bloodstream and travels throughout the body and comes across glucose. The key role insulin has is to help glucose to get inside the cells.

For this to happen, insulin must affix itself to the cell's receptor. When this happens, the cell's membrane will open up, so the glucose can enter. The cell then uses the glucose for its fuel source.

However, for this process to work as it should – you must be in good health.

Should the process fail, the glucose will accumulate in the bloodstream, and the cell won't get the fuel it needs.

This is where diabetes comes about! The lack of a functioning glucose-insulin system

Most people are aware of the two key kinds of diabetes:

- Type 1
- Type 2

Of these, 90 percent of all diabetics are type 2.

Chapter 8: What You Can Do To Reverse Your Diabetes Naturally

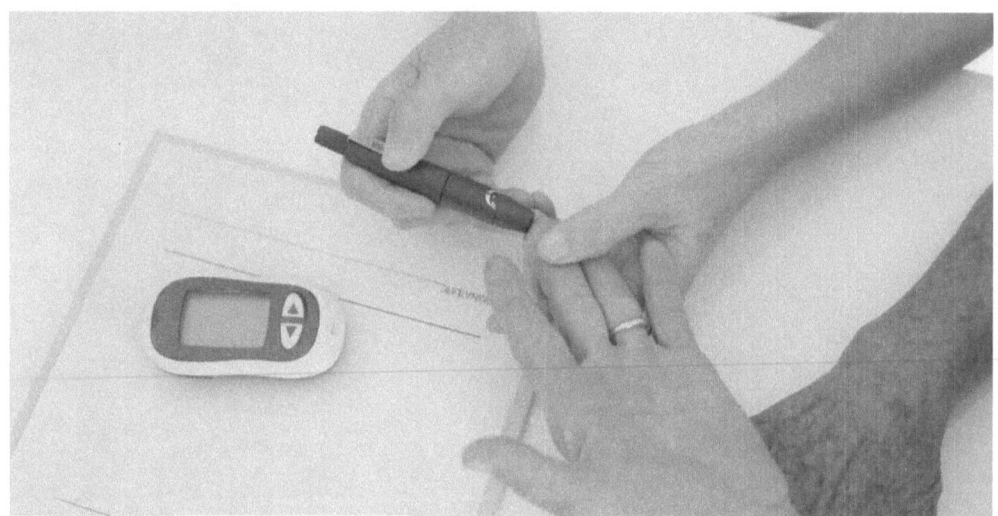

It may surprise you to know that you don't have to always take medications or insulin injections to control your diabetes, especially if you're a type 2 diabetic.

Granted, type 1 diabetics must always use insulin, but there are still natural ways in which people can treat their condition and live a healthy, long life.

Wouldn't it be nice to use a cheaper method of treatment instead of paying the drug companies $10,000+ for your medication? What can you do?

10 Ways To Naturally Treat Diabetes (Preventing and Reversing It In Some Cases)

Take Preventive Measures

A key way to decrease the chance of becoming diabetic is to maintain control over your weight.

About 80 percent of people who are type 2 diabetic are overweight/obese. It's believed obesity causes insulin resistance. Insulin resistance will cause pre-diabetes and type 2 diabetes.

Healthy Diet

Once you've been told that you're diabetic, it's time to take control over your diet. The diet is the key to living healthy with diabetes and naturally reversing it (only if you have type 2 diabetes).

The kind of diet you follow will have a huge impact on your blood sugar levels such as sugar and carbohydrate consumption, as foods with these ingredients are turned into simple sugars known as glucose. Glucose is then released into the body by way of the blood.

The pancreas' beta cells then produce the insulin hormone, which is in charge of getting rid of the glucose and sending to various bodily cells.

The cells need glucose to fuel the body, giving it the energy needed to make it through the day-to-day rigors of life. It's not uncommon for diabetics to suffer from weakness and lethargy because of this very reason.

Since the body isn't using insulin like it needs to be – either through the lack of producing enough or insulin resistance – the glucose stays in the blood and the cells starve from the lack of fuel.

Again, sugar and carbohydrates affect your blood sugar levels, which is why you need to be mindful of any food with them in them – think potatoes, sweet potatoes, cakes, candy, cookies, etc.

The first thing you'll need to do is eliminate refined carbohydrates and simple sugars from your diet. Be sure to eliminate white bread, white pasta and white rice from your diet too since these are also made of refined grains. They also don't have any nutritional value to them and cause blood sugar levels to increase significantly quickly.

They have nothing – like fiber – that allows the body to hold onto them and keep you fuller longer and maintain a steady blood sugar level.

Rather than eating foods with refined carbs, go with complex carbohydrates that ensure the body slowly digests them and can control the blood sugar levels and stop the spikes in blood glucose.

If you're going to reverse your diabetes, you also need to reduce your sugar consumption intake. Sugar plays a huge role in blood sugar levels, which is why it's so important to reduce how much sugar you take in.

Add Fiber

Another way to naturally reverse your diabetes is to add fiber to it. Fiber can help in the slow the digestion process down, which reduces the chances of spikes in blood sugar.

Along with fiber, you need to add in complex carbohydrates (as noted above). Some great sources of fiber include vegetables, fruits, beans and legumes.

Soluble fiber is seen in many different types of food, and once consumed and combined with water, becomes gel-like. This gel-like substance slows down how quickly it goes through the digestive tract, which allows for the control over blood sugar levels.

Fiber is also necessary for any weight loss routine you take up. Fiber will keep you fuller for longer, which means you won't overeat. This is a good thing for diabetics, as most of them are overweight or obese.

The fiber will help in reducing their appetite, allowing them to lose weight while also controlling their blood sugar levels.

Add Cinnamon

Several compounds have proven themselves to reduce blood sugar levels because they help the cells to allow in glucose and properly use the blood sugar. Cinnamon is one such compound. You can use it in all kinds of foods such as cinnamon apples with peanut butter.

Exercise and Workout Routines

High sugar levels can be reduced by adding in exercise to your daily activities. Not only is diet helpful in reducing blood sugar levels, but exercise is key too.

There are all kinds of health benefits to exercise; but, most especially, it's good for your mind, body and soul. People who have diabetes can benefit even further by improving the cells' sensitivity to insulin, which ensures glucose can move into the cells like needed.

As with any exercise program, you need to talk with your doctor to ensure you can do the exercises you want to do. Diabetics are often advised to avoid certain exercises due to complication they may have suffered such as vision or foot problems.

Avoid Saturated Fats or Trans Fat Foods

Be sure to dramatically decrease or stop eating foods that have saturated or trans fats in them. Trans fats, which can be found in foods like margarine, are not good for anybody – diabetics and non-diabetics. Saturated fats can raise the chances of developing heart disease, and diabetics are at an even higher risk of developing heart disease.

Besides the increased chance of developing heart disease, saturated fats can cause insulin resistance, which means who is not diabetic could become pre-diabetic or type 2 diabetic.

Saturated fats are found in foods such as high-fat dairy products, red meats, etc. Make sure to use healthy fats (polyunsaturated and monounsaturated fats) in your diets, which can be found in flaxseed oil, olive oil, olives, cold water fish, seeds, nuts and more.

These minute changes can play a huge role in fighting your

diabetes. **Get Control Over Stress**

It's important to get control over stress, as it can increase your blood sugar levels and cause the body to release stress hormones. Another reason stress is bad for the body in that it can cause you to overeat, lack the will to exercise and more. Diabetics who lower their stress levels have also been able to reduce their blood sugar level.

Create a stress management plan that allows you to focus on the good things in your life – not the stressful ones.

Use Nutritional Supplements

Nutritional supplements can also help you naturally reverse diabetes, as you're taking in more vitamins and minerals your body needs to be healthy.

They work to decrease the chances of suffering from diabetic illnesses such as eye disease, heart disease and nerve damage. They also help to increase insulin sensitivity and reduce your blood sugar level.

Eat Smaller Meals

A key way to avoid the spikes in blood sugar levels is to increase how often you eat and lower how much you consume at that time. Rather than eating the normal two to three big meals – breakfast, lunch and dinner – eat smaller meals at these times and have a mid-day and mid-afternoon snacks to round out your meals.

Change Your Mindset

The reality is that naturally reversing your diabetes begins by changing your mind and life. If you want to be healthy, you need to take a real interest in your health. You must utilize all the information doctors have been telling you and take back your health.

Be open to the idea of using alternative therapies to control your diabetes. Yes, much of it is going to be trial and error, but you rest assured that the answers you are given will help you to control what you're currently dealing with.

Bear in mind that controlling your diabetes is great, but certain foods and medications, stress and more can affect your blood sugar levels significantly.

By being aware of this, you can understand the little bumps in the road and overcome the setbacks a little easier. Don't allow the setbacks to thwart your attempts to live a healthier life as a diabetic.

If you want to overcome your disease and live with it, you need first to accept it!

Conclusion

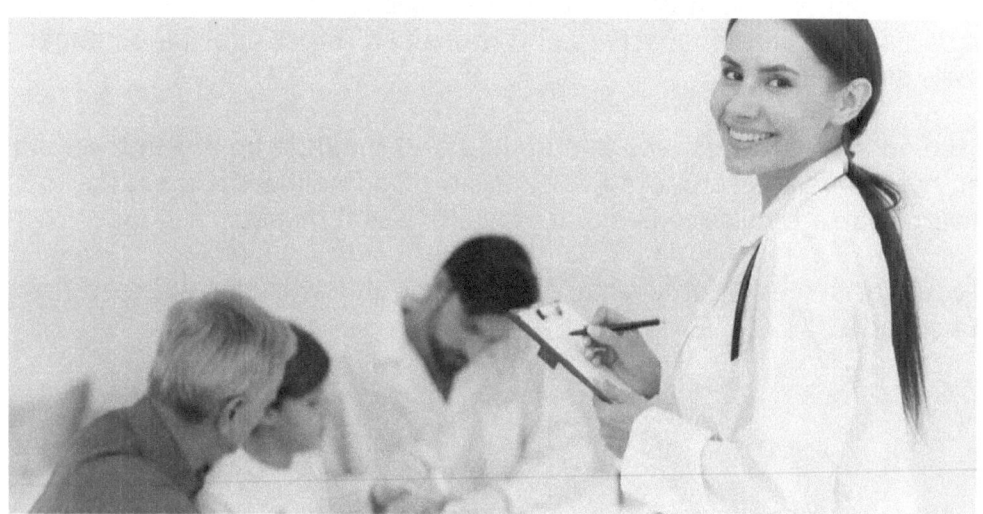

With diabetes so rampant in the world, you or someone you know, and love has it and may not even know it.

It's not just a national health crisis but a global one. If someone in your family has it, you may be worried that you'll be predisposed to it.

If you know that a family member has it, there are things you can do to mitigate your chances of developing it.

And, if you already have diabetes, you may be wondering if it's a death sentence.

You don't have to just accept your lot in life. The choices you make will have a huge effect on whether or not you get the disease and how you live with it if you already have it.

By making some smart decisions and taking the appropriate actions, you can live with diabetes without medications.

Yes, a person who has a family history of diabetes – be it type 1 or type 2 – does have an increased chance of being diagnosed with it. Just because someone in your family has it doesn't mean you will.

Evidence has shown that the best way to stop diabetes, manage it and potentially reverse it is changing how you eat and get in more exercise – not medical treatments.

What's Diabetes Once More?

Remember, diabetes is the result of when the body is unable to use glucose properly. It starts when sugar or glucose enters into the bloodstream after the digestive system breaks down food, and the pancreas releases the insulin hormone. The insulin tells the cells that it needs to absorb the sugar in the bloodstream and use it for fuel.

When a person has diabetes, it means the process isn't functioning as it should be. Some people may find that their pancreas isn't working right and unable to produce the amount of insulin needed.

A lack of this insulin means the cells can't take in sugar. For others, it could be that the body is producing insulin, but the cells cannot respond to the process.

In either case, the body is unable to use sugar as it should. The sugar continues milling around the bloodstream, accumulating. When this happens, they interact with proteins that lead to the development of advanced glycation end products (or AGEs).

These are devastating on the body, damaging all parts of the body:

- Eyes
- Nerves
- Kidneys
- Arteries
- Brain

A person with diabetes may experience an array of diabetes-related complications such as:

- Arteriosclerosis
- Cataracts
- Kidney failure
- Alzheimer's

Diabetes' Genetic Factor

Scientists are in agreement that genetics does play a role in type 1 and type 2 diabetes, but it's just one factor. Identical twin studies were done for type 1 diabetes.

In half of the subjects, both twins developed type 1 diabetes. Researchers feel breastfeeding, environmental factors and viruses had an effect on the genetic disposition.

However, with type 2 diabetes, family has a huge role in developing the disease. And, even though family does have a role in it, it's not sure if genes are a factor.

The key factor behind type 2 diabetes is weight – overweight and obesity. Yes, genetics do play a part in obesity, but family lifestyles and food choices play an even bigger role.

If one were to break the cycle of bad habits, it would mean a break in the diabetes cycle. Evidence suggests that a person has the power to determine if they allow the disease to control them or them control it.

The World Health Organization (WHO) said healthy lifestyle choices could reduce diabetes progression by nearly 60 percent. And, this would also break the need for medications by 30 percent.

You Have The Power To Control Your Diabetes

The best choice you can make in your life is to instill healthy lifestyle changes such as eating better and getting more exercise. Why is that?

When you exercise, the cells use glucose for its fuel. Since they need fuel, the cells can respond better to insulin, allowing them to consume much of the glucose that's accumulated in the blood.

Various studies have shown that high-intensity exercise – even just 10 minutes of exercise – can have a significant impact on the body's ability to be more sensitive to insulin. A look at eight studies show that intense exercise can decrease blood sugar levels for up to three days afterward.

The evidence is even more notable with dieting.

When you consume a lot of sugar and carbs, the body has to generate a plethora of insulin to handle the excess glucose. Due to the amount of strain the body has had put about it, it reacts in one of two ways – stops producing insulin or doesn't respond to the amount produced.

By changing how and what you eat, you can change how the body handles sugar. Without a lot of sugar being consumed, the body can handle what it already has, which means it responds healthily.

There is a lot of research that proves this point. In one study, obese, type 2 diabetic patients underwent significant changes after going on a low-carb diet. Blood sugar levels went back to normal, and they had a 75 percent increase in hormone insulin response.

Due to the amount of research done on diabetes and low-carb diets, many health care professionals have changed how they dealt with diabetic patients. In fact, many doctors and nutritionists have advised patients to do a low-carb diet to get control over their diabetes.

Diabetic Clarity

INFORM, PREVENT, AND MAINTAIN

www.ingramcontent.com/pod-product-compliance
Lightning Source LLC
Chambersburg PA
CBHW030530220526
45463CB00007B/2776